THE BIG BOOK OF JUICE FAST CLEANSE AND DETOX RECIPES

Discover the Secrets of
"Top 50" Best Green Juice Fasting Recipes for Quick Weight Loss, Looking Younger & Boosting Your Stamina

RAVI KISHORE

Text Copyright & Disclaimer © 2013

By: *Ravi Kishore*

All rights reserved. Without limiting the rights under copyright reserved above, no part of the publication may be reproduce, stored in or introduce into a archival system, transferred or transmitted in any form or by any means (electronic, mechanical photocopying, recording or otherwise) without the prior permission of both owner and publisher of this book.

This publication contains the opinions and ideas of its author. it is intended to provide informative material on the subject addressed in the publication. It is sold with the understanding that the author and the publisher are not engaged in rendering medical, health, physiological or any other kind of personal professional services. If the reader requires personal medical, health or other advice/assistance, a competent professional should be consulted.

The author and publisher specifically disclaim all responsibility, loss, or risk, personal or otherwise, that is incurred as a consequence, directly or indirectly, of the use and application of any of the content of this book.

TABLE OF CONTENTS

JUICE FASTING DETOX AND CLEANSING 11

"What exactly is a Juice Fast?" 11

DOES JUICE FASTING HELP YOU TO SHED UNWANTED POUNDS? 12

Why juice fasting is so popular among celebrities and medical professionals: Is juice fasting safe for everyone? 13

STILL CONFUSED: CAN YOU PARTICIPATE IN A "JUICE FASTING" PROGRAM? 15

WANT TO KNOW MORE BENEFITS? 16

TO SUCCEED IS ANY PREPARATION/ PLANNING REQUIRED BEFORE "JUICE FASTING?" 19

PRIOR TO STARTING THE "JUICE FASTING", DETERMINE IF YOUR BODY REQUIRES ANY PREPARATIONS. 22

You want to maintain optimal health while fasting. Don't avoid these instructions & recommendations: 24

HOW DO YOU FEEL? YES, EXPECT PHYSICAL & EMOTIONAL CHANGES BEFORE AND AFTER FASTING 26

SOME QUICK TIPS TO MAKE YOUR JUICE FASTING HEALTHY AND SAFE 29

HOW YOU CORRELATE "JUICE FASTING" WITH "WEIGHT LOSS" 32

IS YOUR WEIGHT LOSS SAFE WITH JUICE FASTING? 33

WHAT ARE THE BEST FRUITS & VEGETABLES FOR WEIGHT LOSS? 34

MYRIAD OF NUTRIENTS THE BODY REQUIRES TO ACHIEVE WEIGHT LOSS GOALS 37

IF YOU ARE A BEGINNER: START A 3-DAY JUICE FASTING CHALLENGE FOR "WEIGHT LOSS" 40

YOU ARE AN EXPERT: HOW TO START YOUR "7 DAY FASTING" CHALLENGE: 43

HOW TO ENSURE THE SUCCESS OF THE FAST: 45

CLEANSING AND DETOXIFICATION WITH JUICING 46

WHICH FRESH JUICES ARE BEST FOR A JUICE FAST 47

JUICE FASTING RECIPES 48

CLEANSING AND DETOXIFICATION RECIPES 48

   CARROT CUCUMBER ZINGER 48

   BROCCOLI SUNRISE 50

   KALE MORNING GLORY 52

MANGO SWEET SURRENDER JUICE	54
FRUITY WATERCRESS JUICE	56
FRUITY FENNEL JUICE	58
GREAT GUAVA JUICE	60
SWEET RADISH JUICE	62
VEGETABLE CILANTRO JUICE	64
FRUITY NUTMEG ELIXIR	66
EASY LIME JUICE	68
CABBAGE JUICE RECIPE	70
STAR FRUIT BREEZE	72
ASPARAGUS DETOX JUICE	74
CUCUMBER APPLE DETOX JUICE	76
HAWAIIAN GINGER ROOT DELIGHT	78
TOMATO JUICE DETOX	80
BLUEBERRY CANTALOUPE JUICE	82
FRUITY ORANGE CHIA JUICE	84
STRAWBERRY KIWI JUICE RECIPE	86

- *CELERY DETOX JUICE RECIPE* 88
- *FRUITY WATERMELON JUICE RECIPE* 90
- *COLLARD GREENS JUICE* 92
- *ONION DETOX JUICE* 94
- *RHUBARB JUICE DETOX* 96

WEIGHT LOSS JUICING RECIPES 98

- *UNBEATABLE JUICE* 98
- *CAULIFLOWER PIZZA JUICE RECIPE* 100
- *PEPPER JUICE RECIPE* 102
- *ZUCCHINI JUICE* 104
- *ORANGE LETTUCE JUICE* 106
- *EGGPLANT ORANGE JUICE* 108
- *BLACKBERRY BLEND* 110
- *PAPAYA JUICE RECIPE* 112
- *GRAPE BLEND* 114
- *CELTUCE JUICE BLEND* 116
- *SPICY CHILI JUICE RECIPE* 118

- CRENSHAW MELON JUICE 120
- VEGGIE APPLE BREEZE 122
- CANTALOUPE JUICE RECIPE 124
- DANDELION DELIGHT 126
- BOLD LEMON JUICE RECIPE... 128
- SWEET PEAR JUICE 130
- GRAPEFRUIT JUICE 132
- PINEAPPLE PASSION JUICE.. 134
- PERFECT PARSNIP JUICE 136
- ARTICHOKE VEGETABLE DELIGHT 138
- REFRESHING MINT JUICE 140
- SWEET POTATO JUICE RECIPE... 142
- TENDER GARLIC JUICE 144
- PLUM JUICE 146

CHOOSING THE BEST JUICER 148

SELECTING THE JUICER 150

HELPFUL TIPS FOR PURCHASING A JUICER.......................151

TOP 10 JUICERS 152

BREVILLE BJE200XL COMPACT JUICE FOUNTAIN 700-WATT JUICE EXTRACTOR 152

HAMILTON BEACH BIG MOUTH JUICE EXTRACTOR 67650 152

BREVILLE 800JEXL JUICE FOUNTAIN ELITE 1000-WATT JUICE EXTRACTOR 153

BREVILLE BJE510XL JUICE FOUNTAIN MULTI-SPEED 900-WATT JUICER 153

BREVILLE JE98XL JUICE FOUNTAIN PLUS 850-WATT JUICE EXTRACTOR 154

OMEGA J8006 NUTRITION CENTER JUICER - BLACK AND CHROME 154

OMEGA J8004 NUTRITION CENTER COMMERCIAL MASTICATING JUICER, WHITE 155

BLACK & DECKER JE2200B 400-WATT FRUIT AND VEGETABLE JUICE EXTRACTOR WITH CUSTOM JUICE CUP 155

TRIBEST CS-1000 CITRISTAR CITRUS JUICER 156

WARING PRO JEX328 HEALTH JUICE EXTRACTOR 156

Juice fasting Detox and Cleansing

You've probably already heard that a juice fast was discovered for mind/body wellness, body detox, and weight loss but probably wanted to know,

"What exactly is a Juice Fast?"

Juice fasts are becoming a popular remedy to help cut down on fat, calories, and to help people lose weight. Juice fasting, also referred to as "juice cleansing," is a detox diet that requires individuals to drink healthy juices to obtain nutrition. While completely abstaining from eating food, dieters use this fasting method to eliminate the body of toxins and excess fat. Unlike diets based on restricting certain fatty foods or requiring the ingestion of supplements, juice fasts are an all-natural alternative to help shed extra pounds. Encouraging the consumption of healthy foods, Juice fasts supplement a low-calorie diet with fruits, vegetables, and legumes that contain liquids. Dietary plans and supplements effectively assist in losing weight, but they also can be harmful. Most dietary plans are harmful because they strip the body of important nutrients needed to burn fat.

Does juice fasting help you to shed unwanted pounds?

As one of the hottest trends in the weight loss industry, juice fasting is popular for its ability to remove excess fat quickly. However, the question remains: does juice fasting help to shed unwanted pounds? For people who are looking to lose weight quickly, juice fasting can assist in achieving fast results. Many individuals who have utilized this method for weight loss have reported losing an average of one pound a day. While juice fasting makes a great start to a weight loss regimen, it is recommended to avoid foods that are high in concentrated carbohydrates after fasting. Juice fasting causes the loss of fat, lean muscle, and water weight because the body does not receive a sufficient amount of calories. When using a juice cleanse, the body improves its absorption of nutrients because the colon walls become free of impacted feces. Returning to high calorie enriched foods after fasting will only produce weight gain instead of continued loss. In determining if juice fasting works, the experts mostly agree that the answer is yes.

Why juice fasting is so popular among celebrities and medical professionals: Is juice fasting safe for everyone?

Most health conscious individuals will want to adhere to the safest practices when attempting a juice fast. While most doctors agree that going on a juice fast will not cause any harm, they also recommend seeing a physician to confirm that you are healthy enough to handle the detox. Another recommendation is to eat a nutrient rich diet a month before beginning a juice fast. When taking into account the current state of health, there are many people who should not participate in a juice fasting regimen. They are listed here:

- Women who are pregnant or nursing
- Diabetics
- Epileptics
- Those suffering from eating disorders
- Those who have a terminal disease
- Those who suffer from hyperglycemia
- Those who have recently undergone surgery
- Those who are afflicted with liver or kidney disease
- Those who have low blood pressure

- People who take prescription drugs daily should consult a doctor as they may not be eligible to participate in some form of a juice fasting regimen.

Still confused: Can you participate in a "JUICE FASTING" program?

Almost anyone over the age of 18 can utilize the health benefits of a juice fast. Since health is a determining factor, juice fasting should be attempted by people who do not suffer from any major complications. The condition of a person's body and mind can have positive or negative effects on the outcome of fasting. Those suffering from cancer, chronic pain, depression, severe infections, arthritis, or autoimmune diseases can speak to their doctor to see if they can go on a juice fast. Many people with these afflictions have used a juice cleansing to help treat their ailments.

Juice fasts not only "cleanse" your body of pollutants, toxins, and food which are laced with preservatives but also help to reset physiological processes and help you lose weight at the same time.

Want to know more benefits?

Unlike some popular diets, juicing supplies the body with many vitamins and minerals. These nutrients cleanse the body, repair the immune system, aid in maintaining proper digestion, and reset physiological processes that have been riddled with pollutants. At the end of a fasting period, dieters can expect to gain many of the health benefits listed here:

- Inducing rapid weight loss, juice fasting places the body in a homeostatic state which quickly burns off fat and calories. Through the process of cleansing, toxins that would normally disrupt various functions in the body are freed up such as the liver, which will begin to burn off fat at an accelerated rate. A juice fast rejuvenates the digestive organs and glands, which contributes to efficient food digestion and less stored food within the body.

- Boosting the immune system, a juice fasting detox positively assists in reversing the effects of a poor diet. Juice cleansings help to eliminate transformed fatty acids, excess body fat, and impacted mucus in the bowels as well as toxins. Allowing the body to focus on total rejuvenation, juice cleansings do not need digestive energy from the body; instead, the body uses these nutrients to increase the production of Lymphocytes which ultimately attack anything harmful found in the body like carcinogens.

- In the brain, juice cleanses have been known to increase neuro-transmissions, improve cognitive functions, and decrease nervousness. Stimulating regeneration in the mind, juice fasting can give a feeling of strength over the needs of the body, which can lead to stronger immune and belief systems. Since the brain works on a chemical level, it must be properly oxygenated. Flushing out the toxins that have crossed the blood/brain barrier thereby enhances intellectual processes.

- Increasing vitality and energy. The juice fasting method helps to restore the body to optimal health. The essential nutrients found in fresh produce quickly travels throughout the vital organs when fasting. They promptly deliver vital nutrients, enzymes, and trace elements directly to the nervous system and major functioning organs resulting in a metabolic energy increase that will eventually flush out toxins in the cellular tissues and mucous from the lymph nodes.

- In the digestive system, juice cleanses loosen up old, hardened fecal matter located in the intestines. Upon the completion of the fast, dieters will flush out and eliminate the fecal matter along with pollutants that have been inside the body for years. Improving digestion contributes to overall body and immune health. Less undigested food that sits in the digestive tract means more energy.

To succeed is any preparation/ planning required before "JUICE FASTING?"

To succeed on a juice fast, proper planning and preparations must be implemented prior to starting the detox. While juice fasting is efficient in cleansing vital organs and strengthening the immune system, improper planning before doing a fast can have adverse effects. Severe dehydration and malnutrition can negatively impact the health of those participating in this cleansing regimen. By regulating and planning for juice supplements the outcome of the fast can be a successful one. Here is a list of preparations to make note of before beginning a juice diet.

- Organize and plan for the fast by writing down vital instructions on a piece of paper. Plan a schedule and gather the appropriate amount of juice recipes needed while on the juice fast. This is important because once fasting begins it will help serve as a reminder. Having the recipes on hand will also make it easy to switch between varying tastes.

- For those of you who do not already own a juicer, go and purchase one online or at a local appliance store. There is a significant difference between a blender and a juicer. While a blender is not capable of properly breaking down all of the fibers in the juice, a juicer completely separates all the juice from the fibers, resulting in a thin, smooth drink.

- Stock up on a variety of organic fruits, vegetables, and legumes that can be juiced. Buy produce that is bright and colorful as this signifies a greater concentration of vitamins and minerals. Produce that should not be juiced are apricots, avocados, bananas, coconuts, cantaloupes, and peaches. Juices made with these fruits will be thick, as the juices of these fruits are unable to be separated from the fiber of the plant.

- Create your own blends of healthy juices and drink them in place of meals and snacks. Do not drink bottled juice from the grocery store because they are less healthy and lack the live enzymes that are present in fresh juice. Fresh vegetable and fruit juices have high amounts of vitamins and minerals. Carrots, green peppers, cucumbers, spinach, and sprouts are great vegetables for juicing.

- It is recommended to drink between 32 and 64 oz. of juice daily. Continue to use the juice fast for three to thirty days. Try to start off small and work up to a longer fast. Fasting takes a toll on the body, so it is best to ease the body into fasting a couple days at a time. As the body adjusts to the juice fasting, dieters can extend the fast as needed.

- There are several benefits to drinking water while on a juice fast. Water plays an essential part in the transportation and digestion of nutrients throughout the body. Alternating between cups of water and cups of juice will help to flush out impurities in the system. It is recommended to drink at least one cup of water in the morning while on a juice fast.

Break the fasting by slowly easing into solid food. The first day off the juice fast, eat a few pieces of fresh fruit. On the second day, consume fruit and add a light vegetable soup to the menu. Finally, on the third day, eat fruits, vegetables, and a light dinner. Do not overwhelm the body by eating high fat sugary snacks or any animal by-products right away.

Prior to starting the "juice fasting", determine if your body requires any preparations.

To succeed on a juice fast, proper planning and preparations must be implemented prior to starting the detox. Going directly from a diet packed full of junk foods straight into fasting can cause some negative side effects. Pushing the body from one extreme to another can send the immune system into shock. By regulating the body before a fast, the host will be able to effectively manage the stress of the fast while maintaining proper nutrition and health.

- Upon deciding to start a fasting, it is best to educate yourself on the fasting technique that you are going to use. Gather all the supplies needed prior to beginning your fast. This will ensure that you are properly prepared, and it will also assist in making you less likely to quit.

- Completely eliminate the use of drugs and foods that are hard to digest from the diet, at the very least, one week before beginning the juice diet. Cut down on sugar, artificial sweeteners, caffeine, alcohol, nicotine, cigarettes, red meat, processed foods, and microwavable meals. Try supplementing these unhealthy items with leafy vegetables, teas, brown rice, and vegetarian soups.

- Start by gradually cutting down on the amount of food consumed in a day. Try implementing more fruits, vegetables, and legumes into regular meals. Remember to slowly eliminate foods that are high in sugar as well. Cutting down on meals a few days before a fasting prepares the body, mind, and stomach for the diet. Do not eat a big supper on the night before the fasting. The less contents that you have in the digestive system before the juice fast, the better.

You want to maintain optimal health while fasting. Don't avoid these instructions & recommendations:

Adhering to the recommendations below can assist in maintaining optimal health while fasting. Since fasting takes a toll on the entire body, it is very crucial to try to implement the least harmful practices. This is the only way to successfully complete the fasting and make it easier to complete. Here is a list of recommendations and instructions to properly begin a juice fasting.

- Drink freshly prepared juice and remember not to store the juice for more than 24 hours. Since juice rapidly loses nutritional and therapeutic value during storage, it is recommended to try to consume all of it before the day is over. If the batch of juice is too big to be consumed at one time, then save it for a couple of hours in a glass jar. Place the lid on it to prevent oxidation.

- Remember to dilute all the fruit juice with 2-4 parts of water. It will help to lessen the consumption of sugar from the fruits. Experts suggest placing 2 cups of the juice blend with ¼ tray of ice cubes. The drink will be frothy, cold, and it will not taste watered down. Vegetable juices do not need to be watered down; instead, they can be consumed right away.

- Try juicing greens in between harder vegetables. The juice will sit at the bottom and will be difficult to pour out of the juicer if you don't. For example, juice a couple of sticks of celery, then some parsley, then add a couple more sticks of celery to get the juicer moving again.

- Don't add more than 25 percent green juice to vegetable juice blends. The mixture can taste bitter and rough and may cause the dieter to vomit it all right back up. Since juices don't stimulate the stomach into releasing acids, it is recommended to use orange and tomato juices that are high in acids. Mix these juices with other, less acidic ones so that they are easily digested.

Break the fasting by slowly easing into solid food. The first day off the juice fasting, eat a few pieces of fresh fruit. On the second day, consume fruit and add a light vegetable soup to the menu. Finally, on the third day, eat fruits, vegetables, and a light dinner. Do not overwhelm the body by eating high fat, sugary snacks or any animal by-products right away.

How do you feel? Yes, expect physical & emotional changes before and after fasting

The number one most frequently asked question when starting to juice fast is, "How will I feel?" This is understandable considering all the physical changes that take place in the body when fasting. Over the long run, juice fasts definitely induce vitality and energy. Due to the differences in each human, the effects of detoxification may vary. Depending on the overall health of the body when starting a fasting, the results can range from slightly sick and bed ridden to highly energized and vibrant.

- The negative physical effects of juice fasting can vary from headaches, nausea, and muscle aches to weakness and muscle cramps. Due to the absence of solid foods, mineral deficits may appear and cause a feeling of fatigue. Blood pressure may also drastically drop, while uric acid levels may rise. None of these symptoms mean that fasting isn't safe, but they do illustrate the body's reaction to severe caloric restriction. During a fast, all the body's energy is used to heal itself, regenerating cells, repairing tissue, and cleansing organs. Experiencing hunger, constipation, and diarrhea as a result of the fast is completely normal. None of these symptoms mean your fast isn't safe, but they do illustrate your body's reaction to severe caloric restriction. Before fasting, the body may be craving some of the foods that have been eliminated from the diet; it is normal to push away those unhealthy cravings with fruit. After fasting, the body will feel rejuvenated and revitalized as all of the toxins and impurities have been flushed from the body.

- The emotional effects of juice fasting vary among individuals. Adopting a positive attitude before the juice fast is very important. These feelings will contribute to calming the nerves as well as the mind. One must demonstrate strong will power to complete a detox. Staying positive provides the well-being needed to go the distance. During the fast, it is normal to be emotional as the absence of solid foods can cause a feeling of vulnerability. After the fast, a heightened sense of clarity and emotional balance usually occur. Feeling accomplished, confident, and proud is also normal after the fasting period. During fasting transitions, people usually question other aspects of their lives and want to make new plans for the future.

Some quick tips to make your juice fasting healthy and safe

Maintaining a healthy body when fasting is the number one objective. While this task can seem difficult, it would be much harder without guidance and direction. It is recommended to gather helpful tips before juice fasting. Any health conscious individuals will want to be properly educated before performing a detox. Here is a list of tips to help dieters safely get through a juice fast.

- Heavy exercise and perspiration is not recommended when fasting. Instead, take up light stretching and walking. When juice fasting, your stamina is not as functional as it normally is. These light exercises can help to keep muscles toned. Take up relaxing activities that will not put too much strain on your body like sun bathing, reading, and sleeping. Remember the purpose of a juice fast is to rejuvenate the body not over exert it.

- Turn off all food temptations so that you will not break the fast by eating. When fasting, try to avoid commercials on the television and the radio. They always advertise food for restaurants, fast food retail chains, and supermarket items. It is recommended to have some delicious pictures hanging around featuring the juice you're going to drink so that the body craves it.

- Having support from family and friends is a great way to ensure the success of a detox. It would be ideal if a friend or family did the cleanse with you as well to provide moral support. Buddies can give each other encouragement, compare notes, share recipes, and help each other through the tough times. They can even take turns making the juice.

- Get motivated by having visual aids available during the fast. If the purpose of the juice fast is to improve your skin complexion then hang up some pictures of yourself with clear skin. For extra motivation use a visual aid of what you'll be giving yourself once the fast is completed. Place them in places that are clearly visible to you throughout the day.

- Colon cleansing is recommended for people going on an extended juice fast. Toxins that are not eliminated through bowel movements get reabsorbed into the system which can cause unnecessary health problems. Talk to a physician to see which colon cleansing method you should use.

- Try juicing greens in between harder vegetables. The juice will sit at the bottom and will be difficult to pour out of the juicer if you don't. For example, juice a couple of sticks of celery, then some parsley, then add a couple more sticks of celery to get the juicer moving again.

- Don't add more than 25 percent green juice to vegetable juices blends. The mixture can taste bitter and rough and may cause the dieter to vomit it all up. Since juices don't stimulate the stomach into releasing acids, it is recommended to use orange and tomato juices that are high in acids. Mix these juices with other less acidic ones so that it is easily digested.

How you correlate "Juice Fasting" with "Weight Loss"

Controlling the body's calorie intake is the common link that connects juice fasting with weight loss.

True weight loss refers to losing fat that is stored inside the body. While Juicing delivers a vast amount of nutrients that break down excess fat, calories, and cholesterol, it naturally induces weight loss. Toxins accumulated in the body inhibit weight loss, damage cells, and make the processes directly linked to weight regulation less efficient. Antioxidants that are present in juicing like vitamin C, vitamin E, and selenium stick to toxins and speed up their elimination from the body. Higher calorie foods such as dairy, meat, and refined carbohydrates are also eliminated during a fast, which reduces the body's calorie intake. Without solid foods in the body, vital organs turn to glycogen and stored fats for energy.

Is your weight loss safe with juice fasting?

Fasting in moderation is considered to be a safe method for cleansing the body of chemicals and toxins.

While it is not recommended to stay on a juice fasting program for longer than a few days when done correctly, this method can assist in weight loss. Fasting for longer than a few days is not recommended as it can induce harmful side effects to the body. Eliminating fiber from the juices during a fasting can also cause side effects such as diarrhea, constipation, and elevated insulin and blood glucose levels. Adding some of the pulp after juicing the fruits and vegetables will allow dieters to receive sufficient amounts of fiber. People with a medical condition should not do a juice fast of any kind without consulting a physician first.

What are the best fruits & vegetables for weight loss?

Fruits and vegetables promote rapid weight loss by providing the body with essential nutrients needed to burn calories and maintain optimum health. Eating low-calorie fruits and vegetables can actually decrease hunger and change negative eating patterns. The more fruits and vegetables that are consumed, the more it will become a personal preference to eat these foods over unhealthy snacks. Here is a list of some of the best vegetables and fruits for weight loss and why.

- Apples can help dieters manage their weight loss and assist in weight management. Low in calories and in dietary fat, apples are an abundant source of fiber, which reduces cholesterol, and they are an appetite suppressant. One single, large apple has more than 5 grams of dietary fiber which is generally found in its skin.

- Pears produce many essential nutrients that can assist in losing weight. High in fiber and low in dietary fat, these fruits have been known to promote hydration and suppress the appetite because of their high water content. A medium-sized pear provides 5.5 grams of fiber. It is recommended to avoid canned pears as they are high in sugar.

- Grapefruit makes the perfect addition to any weight loss program. This fruit is rich in fiber, low in calories, and has tremendous dietary benefits. According to professionals grapefruit cuts down fat and grease built up in the stomach. Grapefruit contains 3.4 grams of fiber which exceeds the daily fiber needs by more than 13%.

- Berries are sweet little fruits that can easily help dieters lose weight. Rich in fiber and antioxidants, berries promote a trim, lean physique. This fiber-rich fruit has been known to improve digestion and is used as an appetite suppressant. Berries are also low-glycemic fruits. This means they have a mild impact on the body's blood sugar which will delay hunger pains. Raspberries alone contain 8 grams of fiber per cup; that's more than a serving of whole-grain pasta.

- Spinach contains many properties that actively assist in weight loss. Rich in fiber, spinach also contains at least 13 phytonutrients called flavonoids. These have antioxidant properties that deliver vitamin C and folates, an important nutrient. Spinach is a very low-calorie veggie that suppresses appetites better than most vegetables.

- Broccoli is a healthy vegetable that makes the perfect addition to any diet. High in antioxidants and low in calories, broccoli fills the stomach with a nutrient-dense fiber that slows the digestive process, providing the feeling of being full. This fiber rich vegetable also provides a low glycemic load which is also beneficial in losing weight.

- Brussels sprouts and cabbages contain many health benefits that contribute to weight loss. Rich in fiber and low in calories, these vegetables provide an excellent source of vitamins and minerals. In addition to being a good source of thiamine, folate, riboflavin, and vitamin E brussels sprouts and cabbages help the digestive system, cellular development, and the nervous system.

- Collard greens and leeks are considered two of the best foods to aid in weight loss. High in fiber and low in calories, these vegetables are packed with amino acids, proteins, and a low glycemic index. Providing 49 calories, collard greens and leeks slow down digestion and reduce hunger cravings.

Myriad of Nutrients the Body Requires to Achieve Weight Loss Goals

Essential vitamins provide adequate nutrition to those on a diet. Commonly found in healthy foods, essential vitamins assist with bodily functions in numerous ways. Maintaining strong bones, healthy red blood cells, and efficient energy conversion are some of the associated benefits. Found in vitamins, minerals, fats, protein, and carbohydrates these additives work in conjunction with one another to deliver all the nutrients needed to achieve weight loss goals.

Vitamins are organic chemical compounds that consist of fat soluble vitamins and water soluble vitamins. While fat soluble nutrients travel throughout the body in fat cells, they are generally stored in the liver and on fatty tissues in the body. These fat soluble nutrients are found in vitamins D, A, K, and E. In contrast, water soluble vitamins cannot be stored in the body; instead, they move through the body in water and exit via the urine or digestive tract.

Minerals are chemical elements that assist with many bodily functions and consist of macro-minerals and trace minerals, which the body needs large quantities of to survive. Macro-minerals are found in magnesium, calcium chloride, phosphorus, potassium, sulfur, and sodium. Micro-nutrients are found in iron, copper, chromium, fluoride, manganese, iodine, molybdenum, selenium, and zinc. The only similarity between them is that the body requires a 100 mg daily dose of each one in order to maintain a healthy state.

Fats are lipids that also assist in many bodily functions. Consuming healthy monounsaturated and polyunsaturated fats while on a diet is essential for losing weight. Used to absorb fat soluble vitamins, fat gives structure to cell walls and stabilizes the body's core temperature. Based on a diet consisting of 2000 calories, it is recommended that a person consume 44-78 grams of fat daily. For the best weight loss results, consume the lower end of the fat grams. To get essential fatty acids, eat oily fish such as mackerel, salmon, sardines, and tuna and plant foods such as olives, nuts, and seeds.

Protein is the most plentiful substance in the body. A healthy diet must contain protein; not only does it induce weight loss, but it also stimulates normal growth and development in the body. Used to repair and build muscle tissue, proteins provide the most important calorie that influences the metabolic rate, which induces weight loss. On a diet consisting of 2000 calories, it is recommended that a person consume 50-175 grams of protein, which is equivalent to 20 to 700 calories of protein a day. Quality protein improves immunity, muscle fitness, and antioxidant function and also helps to sustain muscle during weight loss.

Carbohydrates are starches and sugars that provide energy to the body. Necessary for maintaining health, carbohydrates induce rapid weight loss. Used during digestion, carbs are broken down into glucose which is the body's primary source of energy. On a diet consisting of 2000 calories, it is recommended that a person consume from 225 to 325 grams, which is equivalent to 900 to 1,300 calories a day. Replacing refined grains with whole foods creates a non-digestible carbohydrate called fiber. Fibers suppress hunger because they take longer to chew.

If you are a beginner: Start a 3-day juice fasting challenge for "WEIGHT LOSS"

The Three-Day Juice Challenge is a detoxification and weight-loss regimen that involves consuming only freshly prepared fruit and vegetable juices for three days straight. This system easily sheds pounds, cleanses the body, and eliminates toxins. Highly recommended for people trying this method of weight loss for the first time, and those seeking a light detox, the 3 day challenge makes a great beginning to any weight loss program.

- Before beginning the Three-Day Juice Challenge, it is recommended to consume only raw vegetables and fruit for two days prior to the challenge. During the program, it is important to drink juices made of fresh, raw vegetables, and fruit juices, drink eight glasses of water each day, and don't eat any solid foods.

- Transitioning off of a three-day fast requires a lot of strength as it will be hard to resist the temptations of binge eating. Ease back into dietary routines with small, frequent meals consisting of fresh fruits and salads. Teas and light soups are also okay. The key is to eat light foods that won't apply a lot of stress on the organs and digestive system. Don't eat refined sugars, wheat, or dairy as these foods are too heavy for the digestive tract at this time.

Due to the detoxification process, many dead cells and toxins are rapidly released out of the system in a short time. If fasting is broken in the wrong way, it can cause the elimination of waste to slow down and get absorbed back into the body. Switching the body from being in a cleansing mode back into a normal digestive mode requires patience as the next few days will be just as tough as the fast itself. Here are some strategies to breaking a three-day juice fast.

- Break the juice fast by eating fruits with high water content. Grapefruits contain a high water content, and they are easily digestible.

- Eat raw foods during the transition from fasting. Half of an apple is another option for breaking a fast as it is easily digestible and will restart the metabolism.

- Continue consuming large quantities of broths, herbal teas, and vegetable juices during the transition. Do this for several days to produce nutrition and enzymes in the cells.

You are an Expert: How to start your "7 DAY FASTING" challenge:

The seven day juice fast is a detoxification and weight-loss regimen that involves consuming only freshly prepared fruit and vegetable juices for seven days straight. Unlike the three day challenge this fasting method is recommended for those who have experience with fasting. Experienced individuals will have some idea of the mental and physical tolls a seven day juice fast can present.

- Before beginning the seven day juice fast, it is recommended to refrain from consuming alcohol, coffee, processed foods, and foods that are high in fat. Some of these foods take a long time to digest, which will work negatively when fasting. During the program, drink 32-64 ounces of raw, freshly made juice, along with at least eight glasses of water each day. Don't forget to stay away from solid foods.

- Transitioning off of a seven day fast requires a lot of care as the stomach will be much more sensitive compared to fasting for shorter periods of time. Eat and drink foods that are easily digestible and contain no refined sugars, wheat, or dairy. Teas, broth, and salads are great foods to eat while transitioning off of a seven day fast.

Breaking a seven day fast the wrong way can have many harmful side effects on the body. As the stomach has taken a long break from digestion, it needs anywhere from three to nine days to return back to normal. Here are some strategies to breaking a seven day juice fast.

- Break the juice fast by eating fresh fruit such as watermelon. Watermelon has a high water content making it easily digestible and nutritious.

- Eat fresh vegetable soups to provide nutrition to the body. Do not eat creamy soups. Consume your food slowly and chew food well. Make sure to continue drinking water.

- Three days after the fast, it is safe to consume salads, a baked potato, or a slice of whole grain bread such as manna or brown rice bread.

- On the fourth day, it's safe to add some protein to the diet. Have a small amount of organic chicken, fish, or turkey for dinner. Continue with these foods throughout the rest of the period until digestion returns to normal.

How to ensure the success of the fast:

To succeed on a juice fast, proper planning and preparations must be implemented prior to starting the detox. While this is an effective method for weight loss, it is recommended that you make a plan to ensure the success of the fast.

- Begin by writing down 5-10 reasons why you would like to fast. Then make a list of the pros and cons; if the pros outweigh the cons then you should begin planning for the rest of the juice fast.

- Research and become familiar with the proper methods of juice fasting including helpful tips and advice.

- Next, make a list of the fruits and vegetables you like to eat and then gather the recipes that include these foods. Don't forget to include different recipes for breakfast, lunch, and dinner.

- Now gather all of the things that can provide incentives while fasting like pictures of the outfits you want to wear after you lose the weight. Set them to the side and have them close-by for the times when you feel like giving up the fast.

- Finally, write a list of relaxing activities in which you can take part. Upon fasting, use this list to keep your mind off of eating.

- Get rid of temptations throughout the household. Hide those pictures of apple pies and put those food magazines in the drawers; fasting is a mentally challenging feat as well as a physically difficult one. It is important to surround yourself with pictures and things that will assist you in reaching your goals, not abandoning them.

Cleansing and Detoxification with Juicing

Juicing is a powerful detox that flushes toxins out of the body as a part of an all-natural, self-regulatory cleansing process. People, on average, have at least 5-10 pounds of accumulated toxins in their cells, organs, and tissues. These include pesticides, chemicals, drug residues, food additives, traces of metal, and a long list of toxins found in the environment that people consume on a daily basis. Fortunately with regular juicing, an improvement in the body's ability to detoxify and repair itself on a cellular level is possible.

Which Fresh Juices are best for a Juice Fast

In order to provide the body with a variety of nutrients, consume different juices throughout the day. Drink more raw vegetable juices. This diet is highly recommended and is a natural healing process preferred and followed by people all around the world.

- Green vegetable juices are a good source of nutrients that are low in fiber and sugar, and they can be easily digested.

- Carrot juice is great for boosting the metabolism, which is effective for healing and repairing the body.

- Cranberry juice is helpful in flushing out toxins from the body, which is effective for cleaning out the body.

- Grape juice is great for healing the body. As they are rich in nutrition and anti-oxidants, they effectively stimulate the metabolism as well.

Juice fasting Recipes

Cleansing and Detoxification Recipes

Carrot Cucumber Zinger

Time:	Servings:	Calories:
10 minutes	1	119

The carrot juice is often the most overlooked members of the vegetable blends. Surprisingly sweet and refreshing, carrot juice is one of the most delicious juices available to date. Packed with many vitamins and minerals this juice can be consumed during the morning, noon, or night time.

Ingredients:
- 8 large carrots
- 2 large cucumbers
- 1/2 lemon wedge

Preparation Instructions:

Wash all the ingredients, then peel the skin off of the cucumbers and put them to the side. Place a glass underneath the juicer spout and begin placing the vegetables inside the juicer. Once the glass is full, squeeze the lemon juice into the drink then stir the contents.

Other Health Benefits:

Carrots are rich in dietary fiber, antioxidants and beta carotene. Contributing to vision, bone growth and reproduction, one single carrot offers more than the daily dietary requirement for vitamin A for adults. Made up of various minerals, this vegetable is high in calcium, copper, manganese, potassium and phosphorous. Furthermore, carrots also produce white blood cells that help regulate the immune system by destroying bacteria that cause infections and illnesses. This vegetable has also been made into an antiseptic, cleaning and disinfecting minor scrapes and cuts.

Broccoli Sunrise

Time:	Servings:	Calories:
10 minutes	1	135.2

Broccoli is a popular vegetable that is commonly eaten as a side dish. Surprisingly delicious, this juice has a bold and savory taste. Highly recommended, this vegetable blend is one of the most delicious juices available. This juice can be consumed any time of the day but is best in the morning.

Ingredients:
- 3 celery stalks
- 1 green orange
- 1 broccoli stalk

Preparation Instructions:

Wash all the ingredients, then bring water to boil in a deep saucepan. Now chop up the broccoli florets and place them inside the pot. Leave the vegetable submerged in the boiling water for 1 minute then use a strainer. Place the broccoli in a bowl full of cold water while preparing the rest of the produce. Cut the celery and carrots into pieces then peel and cut the orange. Begin placing the ingredients in one at a time, once it is completely juiced stir it well and drink up.

Other Health Benefits:

Broccoli is a super vegetable that is high in fiber, antioxidants and lutein. Lutein is an antioxidant that is very similar to beta-carotene. As a natural diuretic, broccoli flushes out toxins in the digestive system, assisting in the regulation of bowel movements. Containing many essential vitamins and nutrients, broccoli is a good source of vitamin A, vitamin B6, thiamin, riboflavin, niacin, iron, calcium, and zinc. Broccoli is known as an effective treatment against vision-related diseases, and it has been used in relation to cataracts, and eyesight degeneration. Broccoli has also been used in the treatment against cancer.

Kale Morning Glory

Time:	Servings:	Calories:
5 minutes	1	361.8

Kale, usually found on the side of an entrée, is more than just a garnish, it is great for soups, stews, or salads. As an uncommon juice blend, kale is surprisingly good and tasty. Containing many nutritional benefits, kale comes highly recommended as the super vegetable of the century.

Ingredients:
- 4 stalks of celery
- 2 green apples
- 2 cups of kale
- 1 grapefruit
- 1 cup of blueberries

Preparation Instructions:

Wash all the ingredients, then cut and core the apples. Now peel the grapefruit and cut the pieces so that they can easily fit into the juicer. Chop the kale and celery up and process all the ingredients in the juicer. Once it is completely juiced, stir it well and drink up.

Other Health Benefits:

Kale is a leafy vegetable that is high in antioxidants, and omega 3 fatty acids. Similar to the members of the Brassica family, kale contains phytochemicals that regulate the immune system. Containing many essential vitamins and minerals, kale is a great source of calcium, manganese, copper, iron, potassium, vitamins A, vitamin C and vitamin K. As a source of the natural antioxidant carotenoid and the phytonutrient lutein, Kale flushes out toxins in the body by stimulating the liver detox enzymes. Kale is used in the treatment against cancer, due to this vegetable's high content of antioxidants.

Mango Sweet Surrender Juice

Time:	Servings:	Calories:
10 minutes	1	291.4

Mangos are soft fruits that are eaten raw or in a fruit salad. Popular for their sweet taste and soft texture, mangos are a favorite among many people. Naturally healthy, mangos are a great source of many essential vitamins and minerals. The best time to enjoy this juice is in the morning and afternoon.

Ingredients:
- 2 kiwis
- 1 banana
- 1 orange
- 1 mango

Preparation Instructions:

Wash all the ingredients, then peel the orange, banana, kiwi, and the mango and cut them into sections. Now feed the ingredients to the juicer, when it is finished, stir the juice and drink it immediately.

Other Health Benefits:

Mangos are a sweet fleshy fruit that is high in antioxidants, dietary fiber, and beta-carotene. As a natural diuretic, mangos flush out toxins in the body, cleansing both the digestive system and the urinary tract. This fruit is a good source of nutrients like iron, vitamin A, vitamin C, folic acid, calcium, copper, zinc and phosphorus. Displaying high antibacterial activity, mangos possess anti-inflammatory and Cardio tonic properties that aid in healing many viral diseases. The properties of mangos are also used in viral medications and ointments.

Fruity Watercress Juice

Time:	Servings:	Calories:
10 minutes	1	260.3

Watercress is an edible plant that is commonly found in salads. Known for its peppery and tangy flavor, this juice is a favorite among many. As a high source of vitamins, watercress is a blend that can be consumed during any time of the day.

Ingredients:

    3 oranges
    3 cups of spinach
    2 watercress stalks
    1 stalk of broccoli

Preparation Instructions:

Wash all the ingredients, then bring water to boil in a deep saucepan. Now chop up the broccoli florets and place them inside the pot. Leave the vegetable submerged in the boiling water for 1 minute then use a strainer. Place the broccoli in a bowl full of cold water while preparing the rest of the produce. Cut up the spinach and watercress into small pieces to fit in the juicer. Next peel and cut the oranges into small sections. Begin placing the ingredients in one at a time, once it is completely juiced stir it well and drink up.

Other Health Benefits:

Watercress is a perennial vegetable that is high in protein, antioxidants, and pantothenic acid. Stimulating salivary, gastric secretions, and the regulation of the intestinal tract, watercress flushes out impurities from the body. Full of essential nutrients watercress has folate, protein, copper, riboflavin, manganese, potassium, thiamin, vitamin A, vitamin C, vitamin E, and vitamin B6 in it. Watercress treats and prevents many forms of chronic bronchitis and known to modify bronchial secretions while exerting an expectorant effect. Watercress is also an active treatment against chronic and degenerative diseases.

Fruity Fennel Juice

Time:	Servings:	Calories:
5 minutes	1	341

Fennel is an herb that is commonly used in cooking. Known for its bold and unique flavor, this herb makes one of the tastiest juices. Packed with many vitamins and minerals, fennel juice is great for any time of the day.

Ingredients:
- 2 Comice pears
- 2 medium fennel bulbs

Preparation Instructions:

Wash all the ingredients, then cut and core the Comice pears. Afterwards, chop up the fennel bulbs and begin placing all of the ingredients into the juicer. Once it is finished, mix it for 1 minute to make sure the contents mixed properly.

Other Health Benefits:

Fennel is an herb that is high in dietary fiber, and calcium. The roughage of fennel seeds acts like a laxative, flushing out the bowels stimulating the peristaltic motion of the intestines, thereby helping proper excretion. Containing many healthy nutrients like phosphorus, niacin, iron, magnesium, and copper. Fennel contains carminative properties of aspartic acid that can cure flatulence and expel gasses of the stomach. Fennel also protects the eyes from inflammation and disorders related to aging.

Great Guava Juice

Time:	Servings:	Calories:
5 minutes	1	157.9

Guava is a tropical fruit that is commonly eaten raw or found in fruit salads. Surprisingly sweet and juicy, this little fruit contains many essential vitamins and minerals. Enjoy this all-natural drink anytime of the day.

Ingredients:
- 2 grapefruits
- 1 guava
- 1 kiwi fruit

Preparation Instructions:

Wash all the ingredients, then peel and cut the grapefruits, and the kiwi. Now chop up the guava fruit and place all of the ingredients inside of the juicer. Mix for 45 seconds or until the mixture is smooth.

Other Health Benefits:

Guava is a fruit that is very rich in vitamin C, and fiber. Containing a large amount of astringents, guava loosens up bowels and promotes digestive regularity. As a rich source of nutrients, guava has potassium, copper calcium, iron, magnesium, phosphorus, zinc, vitamin E and vitamin K. Strengthening and toning the digestive system, these nutrients help to flush out toxins and chemicals. Combating free radicals, guava aids in preventing age related chronic diseases, such as rheumatoid arthritis, Alzheimer's, heart disease and cataracts.

Sweet Radish Juice

Time:	Servings:	Calories:
10 minutes	*1*	*133.8*

Radishes are root vegetables that are commonly eaten raw, in garden salads, or in stews. Surprisingly sweet and bold, this juice comes highly recommended. Drink this all-natural mixture throughout the day to gain energy and vitality.

Ingredients:
- 1 apple
- 1 carrot
- 1 beet
- 1 radish
- 1 cabbage leaf

Preparation Instructions:

Wash all the ingredients, then remove the outer skin of the beet with a potato peeler or knife then cut it into small chunky pieces. Next, cut open the apple and remove the core. Then cut off the leaves, stem, and roots of the radish. Chop up the cabbage leaves and begin putting all of the ingredients in the juicer.

Other Health Benefits:

Radishes are red vegetables that are high in dietary fiber, and vitamin C. Stimulating the production of bile, radishes assist in digestion, as well as, liver and gallbladder health. Additionally, radishes contain many essential nutrients like potassium, calcium, iron, phosphorus, copper, zinc, vitamin A, vitamin B, and vitamin K. Radishes purify the blood and raise oxygen levels, which is why it is currently being used to treat jaundice. Many studies have concluded that antioxidants reduce cholesterol levels in the body which reduces the risk of heart problems.

Vegetable Cilantro Juice

Time:	Servings:	Calories:
10 minutes	2	212.3

Cilantro is a flavorful herb that can be found in salads, in stews, and in meals. Delivering a burst of robust flavor, cilantro makes the best juice as it is high in nutrients. The best time to enjoy this juice is in the afternoon and the evening as it may be too hard on the stomach in the morning, especially if fasting.

Ingredients:
- 2 stalks of celery
- 4 beets
- 2 stalks of cilantro
- 1/2 of spinach

Preparation Instructions:

Wash all the ingredients, then remove the skin from the beets and cut into a size that is appropriate for the juicer. Next chop up the celery, cilantro, and spinach to fit into the juicer. Place all of the ingredients in the juicer, and blend for 1 minute until the juice is smooth.

Other Health Benefits:

Cilantro is an herb that is packed with antioxidants, and dietary fiber. Assisting in the production of digestive enzymes, cilantro regulates the body while flushing out toxins in the system. Additionally this juice offers many nutrients folate, iron, manganese, vitamin C, vitamin A and vitamin K. As an anti- inflammatory, cilantro has been used to alleviate symptoms of arthritis. Containing good qualities of alcohol like borneol, cilantro is effective for destroying viruses and germs that cause colds. It has also been known as a natural anti-inflammatory that helps to alleviate the symptoms of arthritis.

Fruity Nutmeg Elixir

Time:	Servings:	Calories:
5 minutes	1	413

Nutmeg is a flavorful spice that is usually cooked into foods and used to garnish desserts. Packed with a sweet sensational taste, this juice is a popular blend used by many. High in nutritional value, nutmeg juice can be enjoyed any time of the day.

Ingredients:
- 4 apples
- 2 parsnips
- 3 teaspoons of nutmeg

Preparation Instructions:

Wash all the ingredients, then cut and core the apples. Chop up the parsnips and add all of the remaining ingredients to the juicer, including the nutmeg. Blend for 1 minute until the juice is smooth and free of produce chunks.

Other Health Benefits:

Nutmeg is a spice that is high in fiber and manganese. Removing excess gas in the intestines, nutmeg relieves irritable bowel syndrome and flatulence. Additionally, this juice is high in many nutrients like calcium and iron. Cleaning out the toxins in the liver, nutmeg is effective in preventing and dissolving kidney stones. Abundant in anti-bacterial properties, nutmeg has been known to clean out the bacteria in the mouth caused by halitosis or bad breath.

Easy lime Juice

Time:	Servings:	Calories:
5 minutes	1	142

Limes are a fruit that is commonly eaten raw, in salads, or squeezed to add flavor to certain foods. Known for its sour taste, this fruit has many health properties. Great for any time of the day this juice is better when it is cold.

Ingredients:
- 4 white grapes
- 1 lime
- 1 liter water
- 8 tablespoons of honey

Preparation Instructions:

Wash all the ingredients, then peel and cut the lime into small chunky pieces. Place all the rest of the ingredients into the juicer and mix for 45 seconds until the mixture is smooth. Add ice cubes and enjoy the taste of this drink immediately.

Other Health Benefits:

Lime is a fruit that is high in citric acid. Stimulating the digestive system and increasing the secretion of digestive juices, like bile and acids, limes also stimulate peristaltic motion. Additionally, this juice is high in many nutrients like vitamin C, vitamin A, potassium, calcium and iron. Limes contain many anti-oxidants, anti-biotic and disinfectant abilities; they also have been used for skin care including rashes, and bruises. Clearing out the excretory system, the acids found in lime wash and clean off the tracts.

Cabbage Juice Recipe

Time:	Servings:	Calories:
5 minutes	1	186.3

Cabbage is a leafy vegetable that is usually eaten in salads and as a side dish. Known for its robust and crunchy flavor, cabbage juice is a favorite blend among many people. High in nutritional value cabbage juice can be enjoyed any time of the day.

Ingredients:
- 3 oranges
- 1/2 of cabbage
- 5 almonds

Preparation Instructions:

Wash all the ingredients, then peel and cut the orange into pieces that can easily fit into the juicer. Chop up the cabbage and then add all of the ingredients to the juicer including the almonds. Mix for 45 seconds, until the mixture is smooth.

Other Health Benefits:

Cabbage is a vegetable that is high in dietary fiber, and vitamin C. Cabbage contains very high levels of fiber which helps retain water and great for the digestive system. Thus, it is a good cure to help with constipation and related problems. Containing many nutritional benefits, cabbage includes protein, thiamin, phosphorus, copper, vitamin A, vitamin B6, folate and magnesium. High in sulphur, cabbage is very effective in fighting against infections. Rich in iodine, cabbage promotes brain function and the nervous system, as well as, keeping the endocrine glands in proper condition.

Star Fruit Breeze

Time:	Servings:	Calories:
10 minutes	1	248.3

Star fruit is a star shaped fruit that is commonly eaten raw, and in fruit salads. Naturally sweet and tart flavored, star fruit makes one of the most delicious tropical juices known to date. This fruit is also high in nutritional value and is great for busy mornings, when a spike in energy could be useful.

Ingredient:
- 6 strawberries
- 2 pears
- 2 oranges
- 1 star fruit

Preparation Instructions:

Wash all the ingredients, then core and cuts the pears, and oranges, into pieces that can easily fit inside of the juicer. Next, chop up the strawberries and the star fruit, as well. Add these ingredients to the juicer and blend for 45 seconds. Once the juice is finished, mix it well before drinking.

Other Health Benefits:

Star fruit is a fruit that is high in dietary fiber, and pantothenic acid. Assisting in the maintenance of the digestive system, this fruit adds bulk and moisture to feces, enabling easy bowel movements. Containing many essential nutrients, this fruit is high in vitamin A, vitamin C, and iron. High in polyphenol antioxidants, star fruit is an effective treatment for respiratory problems, and cardiovascular disease. Given its anti-microbial property, star fruit has been used to treat bacterial infections such as staph, salmonella, and e-Coli.

Asparagus Detox Juice

Time:	Servings:	Calories:
10 minutes	4	47.9

Asparagus, known to many as the aristocratic vegetable, makes the best juice used as a detox. Rich and robust, asparagus juice is one of the most delectable beverages available to date. Packed with many essential vitamins and minerals this juice is best mixed with sweet fruits.

Ingredients:
- 10 stalks of asparagus
- 1 lemon
- 1 tsp olive oil

Preparation Instruction:

Wash all ingredients, then peel the skin off of the lemon. Then place all the ingredients into the juicer, blend for 1 minute until the juices texture is smooth then drink the juice as is or chill for a couple minutes in the freezer.

Other Health Benefits:

Asparagus is high in fiber, proteins and antioxidants. While repairing skin problems, vision problems and the nervous system, asparagus helps the body get rid of waste fast and effectively. Made up of many essential vitamins and minerals like vitamin C, iron, calcium, niacin, copper, and folic acid, asparagus is used to clean out the system. As a natural diuretic, this vegetable flushes out toxins out of the body promoting optimum kidney health. Asparagus contains several antioxidants making it useful in treatments to help reduce tumors and prevent cancer.

Cucumber Apple Detox Juice

Time:	Servings:	Calories:
15 minutes	8	76.1

Cucumbers are a well-known part of a garden salad or sandwich while blending them into a juice is an uncommon practice. Those who have tried this juice say it is simply amazing. Refreshing and sweet, cucumber juice is one of the healthiest blends easily made from home.

Ingredients:

    8 carrots
    4 apples
    1 cucumber
    2 inches of ginger root

Preparation Instructions:

Wash all the ingredients, then chop up the cucumbers and apples into four pieces, remove the apple core, and place the produce to the side. Next cut the ginger root into half pieces. Begin juicing the apple piece first then the carrots ending with the ginger. Refrigerate this drink for a couple of minutes then enjoy.

Other Health Benefits:

Cucumber juice is a diuretic that is high in fiber, protein, and calcium. Contributing to the regulation of the body and blood pressure, cucumbers remove the body waste and toxins. The benefits of cucumbers are mainly found in its skin, which includes vitamins A, C, folic acid, potassium, magnesium, molybdenum, and silica. Containing high alkaline levels, cucumbers regulate the body's blood pH and neutralizes acidity. This vegetable has also been used for diabetic patients since ages. Cucumbers possess a hormone needed by beta cells during insulin production.

Hawaiian Ginger Root Delight

Time:	Servings:	Calories:
10 minutes	2	199.8

Ginger root is commonly found in spice racks. Blending this herb into a juice is usually unheard of, and it comes highly recommended for those who have tried it. Tangy and bold, ginger root is easily made, and it contains many healthy properties.

Ingredients:

    1 pineapple
    2 oranges
    1 inch slice ginger root

Preparation Instructions:

Wash all the ingredients, then place the pineapple on a clean even surface and use a sharp knife to remove the crown and base of the fruit. Next slowly slice the rind off the pineapple. Now cut the pineapple into chunky pieces and set aside. Peel the skin from the oranges and slice each fruit into four sections. Then chop up the ginger root into smaller pieces, as well. Now juice all the ingredients and enjoy.

Other Health Benefits:

Ginger root is a diuretic that is high in antioxidants, protein and calcium. A remedy for travel sickness, nausea, and indigestion, ginger root is excellent for inducing circulation throughout the body. Ginger root contains many vitamins and minerals including vitamin E, vitamin C, vitamin K, potassium, iron, magnesium, phosphorus, sodium, zinc, copper, manganese and selenium. Containing anti-inflammatory properties, ginger root has more than twelve types of anti-oxidants, making it a great treatment for a variety of disorders. This vegetable has also been used to treat rheumatic and inflammatory conditions.

Tomato Juice Detox

Time:	Servings:	Calories:
5 minutes	1	157.4

Tomatoes are an important ingredient commonly found in salads and on sandwiches. While blending them to make a juice is a common practice, these drinks usually come highly recommended for those who have tasted it. Fresh and tasty, tomato juice is excellent for an early morning pick-me up, or an afternoon snack.

Ingredients:
- 2 tomatoes
- 2 carrots
- 2 stalks of celery
- 1/4 onion
- 1/2 of ginger root

Preparation Instructions:

Wash all the ingredients, then chop up the tomatoes, carrots, celery, ginger root and onion into chunky pieces. Begin placing the ingredients into the juicer and blend until the mixture is smooth. Then drink and enjoy.

Other Health Benefits:

Tomatoes are a natural diuretic that is high in antioxidants, and dietary fiber. Assisting the digestive system, and the metabolism, tomatoes stimulate a detoxification function in the liver and lungs. Tomatoes are high in nutrition and vitamin A, vitamin C, vitamin K, and vitamin B6. Tomatoes contain many essential minerals like folate, thiamin, niacin, magnesium, phosphorus and copper. Tomatoes also contain nutrients that help the immune system by destroying the free radicals located in the blood stream that cause damage to cells. This vegetable has also been used to treat heart disease.

Blueberry Cantaloupe Juice

Time:	Servings:	Calories:
10 minutes	*3*	*142.2*

Blueberries are a well-known part of a fruit salad or a parfait. Said to be one of the most delicious juices available to date, blueberry juice is sweet, and juicy. Packed with many vitamins and minerals, this juice can be consumed any time of the day.

Ingredients:

    3 apples
    1 cup of blueberries
    1/2 cantaloupe

Preparation Instructions:

Wash all the ingredients, then peel the apple and remove the core. Next cut the netted skin off of the cantaloupe and begin feeding the fruit to the juicer. Once the juice is finished, add ice and drink immediately.

Other Health Benefits:

Blueberries are a diuretic that is high in antioxidants, dietary fiber, and tannins. Killing bacteria and viruses, blueberries prevent bladder infections and flush out the body. Blueberries contain many nutrients like vitamin A, vitamin C, vitamin E, vitamin K, vitamin B6, as well as, iron, calcium, manganese, phosphorus and copper. Furthermore, blueberries also contain anthocyanin, an antioxidant plant pigment that contributes to its distinctive color. This fruit has also been used to fight diabetes, urinary tract infection, and anti-aging cosmetics.

Fruity Orange Chia Juice

Time:	Servings:	Calories:
10 minutes	2	219.9

Oranges are best eaten raw or blended into a juice. Said to be one of the most popular fruits, orange juices are sweet, and delicious. Packed with many vitamins and minerals, this juice is best in the morning as it delivers lots of energy.

Ingredients:
- 2 oranges
- 2 apples
- 2 carrots
- 1 cup of strawberries
- 2 tbsp of dry chia seeds

Preparation Instructions:

Wash all the ingredients, then peel the rind off the oranges and cut the fruits into four pieces each. Once that is completed slice the apple, core it, and cut it into four parts, as well. Cut the carrot into small pieces and process them in the juicer. Continue adding the remaining ingredients, except for the chia seeds. When the juicing process is completed, then add the chia seeds and stir well for 1 minute.

Other Health Benefits:

Oranges are high in fiber, calcium, and antioxidants. As a natural diuretic, they are great for the digestive system and for relieving constipation. Stimulating the production of white blood cells, oranges aid the immune system and prevents illnesses. Oranges contain many essential vitamins and minerals like iron vitamin B6, folate, potassium, and thiamin. Furthermore, oranges greatly reduce cholesterol due to an alkaloid found in the orange peel. This fruit is also used to treat several other diseases like asthma, arthritis, bronchitis, rheumatism and diabetes.

Strawberry Kiwi Juice recipe

Time:	Servings:	Calories:
5 minutes	4	83.8

Strawberries are known to many as nature's candy. Said to be one of the sweetest fruits, strawberries make the best detox juices as they are very tasty and can be used to satisfy a sugar craving. This juice is healthy and is best consumed in the morning or afternoon.

Ingredients:

    2 apples
    2 cups of strawberries
    1 kiwi

Preparation Instructions:

Wash all of the ingredients, then take a sharp knife and begin cutting off both ends of the kiwi. Now use a spoon to separate the kiwi's skin from the fruit and cut it into quarters. Next, slice open the apple and remove the core from its center. After this is completed, cut the apple into sections and begin placing these pieces into the juicer. Blend the ingredients until the liquid is a smooth texture.

Other Health Benefits:

Strawberries are high in antioxidants, zinc, and dietary fiber. Regulating the digestive system, these fruits can lower blood pressure and prevent overeating. Containing many vitamins and minerals, strawberries deliver Vitamin A, vitamin C, alpha and beta carotene, folate, potassium, and manganese. Enhancing the immune system, strawberries fight against infectious diseases like a cold or flu. Used as a remedy against inflammatory diseases, strawberries have been used to treat asthma, osteoarthritis and atherosclerosis.

Celery Detox Juice recipe

Time:	Servings:	Calories:
5 minutes	*2*	*153.3*

Celery is a crunchy vegetable that is usually found in salads, stews, or eaten raw as a snack. Known for its bold and robust flavor, this juice can deliver enough energy to last the entire day. Celery juice can also be consumed before bed as it contains natural calming agents.

Ingredients:

 5 carrots
 2 stalks of celery
 1 apple
 1/2 broccoli stalk

Preparation Instructions:

Wash all the ingredients, then bring water to boil in a deep saucepan. Now chop up the broccoli florets and place them inside the pot. Leave the vegetable submerged in the boiling water for 1 minute then use a strainer. Place the broccoli in a bowl full of cold water while preparing the rest of the produce. Cut the celery and carrots into pieces, then slice and core the apple. Begin placing the ingredients in one at a time, once it is completely juiced stir it well and drink up.

Other Health Benefits:

Celery is a natural cleanser rich in folic acid, iron and vitamin C. Actively regulating the digestive system, this vegetable softens stools and induces a normalcy of bowel movements. Celery contains many nutritional properties including calcium, magnesium, phosphorus, vitamin A, vitamin B1 and vitamin B2. Enhancing the activity of white blood cells, celery contains coumarin which is a class of antioxidants that have been used to fight cancer. Celery juice also aids in breaking the elimination of urinary and gall bladder stones.

Fruity Watermelon Juice recipe

Time:	Servings:	Calories:
5 minutes	1	118

Watermelons are the perfect addition to fruit salads or eaten raw as a snack. Highly recommended as one of the best tasting drinks available. This fruit juice can be consumed any time of the day, but is the most beneficial in the morning as it delivers lots of energy.

Ingredients:
- 1/8 large watermelon
- 8 strawberries
- 1 apple

Preparation Instructions:

Wash all the ingredients, then use a sharp knife to trim the skin off of the watermelon. Cut the watermelon into small pieces that fit into the juicer. Next slice the apple and take out its core. Begin putting all the ingredients into the juicer and stir once completed.

Other Health Benefits:

Watermelon is a diuretic that is high in antioxidants, fiber and lycopene. Protecting cells against free radicals in the body, lycopene acts like an antioxidant in the body. There are many healthy properties associated with watermelons as they have vitamin A, vitamin C and potassium. Used in the treatment of bladder infections, and to flush out the body, watermelons are one of the best fruits to use in a detox. The antioxidants in watermelons reduce the risk of heart disease, colon cancer and rheumatoid arthritis.

Collard Greens Juice

Time:	Servings:	Calories:
10 minutes	1	52

Collard Greens are a leafy vegetable that is commonly cooked with meals. Collard green juice is rich and robust and is said to be one of the most delectable beverages available to date. Packed with many essential vitamins and minerals, this juice is best after breakfast.

Ingredients:
- 2 stalks of celery
- 1 ginger root
- 1/4 cup of collard greens
- 4 romaine lettuce leaves
- 2 tsp. lemon Juice
- 1 tsp. fennel seed

Preparation Instructions:

Wash all the ingredients, then chop up the celery, ginger root, collard greens and lettuce into chunky pieces. Next, begin placing the vegetables and the lemon juice into the juicer. After the juice is finished, place the fennel seeds in the glass, mix well.

Other Health Benefits:

Collard Greens are high in fiber, proteins and antioxidants. While repairing skin problems,

Vision problems, and the nervous system, collard greens help the body get rid of waste fast and effectively. Made up of many essential vitamins and minerals like vitamin C, iron, calcium, niacin, copper, and folic acid, collard greens are used to clean out the system. As a natural diuretic, this vegetable flushes out toxins out of the body, promoting optimum kidney health. Collard greens contain several antioxidants that help reduce tumors and prevent cancer.

Onion Detox Juice

Time:	Servings:	Calories:
10 minutes	5	112.3

Onions are round vegetables that are usually eaten in salads, on meats and, in rare cases, raw. While blending this vegetable into a juice is usually uncommon, it comes recommended for those who have tried it. Tangy and bold, onion juice is easily made, and it contains many healthy properties.

Ingredients:
- 4 mung bean sprouts
- 3 cups of kale
- 3 carrots
- 3 stalks of celery
- 2 mung bean sprouts
- 2 apples
- 2 pears
- 1 red pepper
- 1 cucumber
- 16 cilantro stems and leaves
- 1/2 onion
- 1 garlic clove

Preparation Instructions:

Wash all the ingredients, use a sharp knife to slice and core the apples, pears and peppers. Now chop up the remaining ingredients and begin to add everything to the juicer. Alternate between ingredients to allow the juicer to blend the juice properly.

Other Health Benefits:

Onions are a natural diuretic that is high in antioxidants, protein and calcium. A remedy for travel sickness, nausea, and indigestion with anti-inflammatory and anti-bacterial properties, onions relieve gastro syndromes. Additionally, onions contain many nutrients like vitamin C, vitamin E, vitamin K, iron, potassium, magnesium, phosphorus, sodium, zinc, copper, manganese and selenium. Preventing the red blood cells from forming clumps, onions are an effective treatment for heart disorders and cardiovascular diseases. This vegetable has also been used to treat anemic conditions, as well.

Rhubarb Juice Detox

Time:	Servings:	Calories:
10 minutes	11	145

Rhubarb is a vegetable that is commonly found in pie fillings, salads, stir-fry's and desserts. While blending them to make a juice is an uncommon practice, these drinks usually come highly recommended for those who have tasted it. Naturally tart and sweet, rhubarb juice is great for any time of the day as a snack or pick-me up.

Ingredients:
- 7 large carrots
- 4 large apples
- 1 stalk of rhubarb
- 1 lb of cranberries

Preparation Instructions:

Wash all the ingredients. Use a sharp knife to cut and core the apples. Trim the ends off of the rhubarb, then discard any leaves. Chop up the carrots and begin adding the ingredients to the juicer. Once the juice is finished add some ice cubes to chill the drink.

Other Health Benefits:

Rhubarb is a vegetable that is high in dietary fiber and vitamin C. Used to stimulate the motility of isolated gallbladder muscle strips, rhubarb is effective in promoting internal health. Additionally, rhubarb contains lots of nutrients like vitamin C, vitamin K, calcium potassium, thiamin, magnesium, and a very good source of dietary fiber. Rhubarb contains many anti-oxidant, anti-inflammatory and anti-allergic activities, it has also been used to treat heart disease.

Weight Loss Juicing Recipes

Unbeatable Juice

Time:	Servings:	Calories:
10 minutes	1	158.1

Beet juice is a dark purplish red juice made from beetroot (Beta Vulgaris). Although it is not a very popular food item, beet juice is one of the tastiest treats Mother Nature has to offer. Packed with many essential vitamins and minerals this juice is best mixed with sweet fruits.

Ingredients:
- 2 carrots
- 1 apple
- 1/2 beet

Preparation Instructions:

Wash all the ingredients, then peel the beets, and apples. Slice out the apple core and begin cutting all of the produce into chunks. Now place all of the ingredients into the juicer, blend for 45 seconds or until the liquid is smooth. Serve chilled.

Other Health Benefits:

Beets are rich in fiber, antioxidants and high complex carbohydrates. Contributing to cardiovascular health, stamina and the stimulation of red blood cells, beets promote regularity in the body. Made up of many essential vitamins and minerals like vitamin C, iron, folic acid, copper, potassium, magnesium and phosphorous, beets are beneficial as a liver tonic and blood builder. Furthermore, beets also assist in the improvement of athletic performance and significantly lowers high blood pressure. In Europe, this vegetable has also been used to treat cancer.

Cauliflower Pizza Juice recipe

Time:	Servings:	Calories:
10 minutes	1	101

Cauliflower is a healthy white food that is commonly found in a crunchy salad, or slaw. While blending them in a juice are an uncommon practice, those who have tried it, have complimented its unique flavor. Robust and crunchy, cauliflower juice are great for lunch time, or dinner time.

Ingredients:
    1 cauliflower head
    1 bunch of spinach
    1 lime

Preparation Instructions:

Wash all the ingredients, then peel the rind off the lime and cut it into four sections. Now chop up the spinach and the cauliflower into small pieces that fit into the juicer. Stir the juice afterward to make sure all the ingredients blended properly.

Other Health Benefits:

Cauliflower is a cruciferous vegetable high in protein, dietary fiber, and phytochemicals called glucosinolates. Regulating the body's detoxification enzymes with these chemicals, cauliflower effectively cleanses out the body.

Containing many nutrients like vitamin C, vitamin K, vitamin B6, niacin, folate, magnesium, and phosphorus, cauliflower is fat free and low in calories. Cauliflower is a great source of alkaline which purifies the blood.

Pepper Juice recipe

Time:	Servings:	Calories:
10 minutes	12	148.6

Peppers are flavorful vegetables most commonly used to spice up food, in salads, or as a garnish. Said to be one of the most sensational drinks, pepper juice is robust and spicy. Great for an afternoon pick-me up or nighttime banquet.

Ingredients:
- 36 carrots
- 16 stalks of celery
- 4 bell peppers
- 4 apples
- 4 mini cucumbers

Preparation Instructions:

First wash all the ingredients. Now slice open the apple, core its center, and cut the apple into sections. Next, remove the center of the peppers and cut it into slithers. Chop up the celery, carrots and cucumbers, as well, then begin feeding the pieces into the juicer. Stir afterward to make sure all the ingredients blended properly and store all unused juice.

Other Health Benefits:

Peppers are a spice that is high in dietary fiber, Iron, and capsaicin. Capsaicin causes a shift in oxidation of carbohydrates to fat oxidation, which decreases the appetite. Peppers contain many vital nutrients like niacin, riboflavin, potassium, magnesium, vitamin E, vitamin K, vitamin A, vitamin C, vitamin B6 and manganese. Consuming peppers increase the metabolism, encouraging the body to burn calories rapidly. The capsaicin in this vegetable has also been linked to pain relieving qualities, as well.

Zucchini Juice

Time:	Servings:	Calories:
5 minutes	1	151.1

Zucchini juice is often the most overlooked members of the fruit blends. Surprisingly tangy and bold, zucchini juice is one of the most delicious juices available to date. Packed with many vitamins and minerals, this juice can be consumed anytime of the day.

Ingredients:
- 1 cup butternut squash
- 1 cup of zucchini
- 1 tbsp of honey

Preparation Instructions:

Wash all the ingredients, then trim the skin off of the zucchini if it has been coated with produce wax. Zucchinis that are not covered in this material allow for the entire vegetable to be thrown in the juicer. Next peel the butternut squash and cut it into strips, and place these ingredients into the juicer. Mix the juice thoroughly, to make sure the veggies are juiced to perfection.

Other Health Benefits:

Zucchini is rich in antioxidants, and dietary fiber. Containing natural inflammatory properties, this vegetable helps prevent bruising in the body and asthma. Made up of many minerals, this fruit is high in protein, thiamin, niacin, copper, vitamin C, vitamin K, vitamin B6 and folate. Additionally, zucchini also produce white blood cells which help regulate the immune system by destroying bacteria that cause infection and illnesses. This fruit has also been made into an antiseptic cleaning and disinfecting minor scrapes and cuts.

Orange Lettuce Juice

Time:	Servings:	Calories:
5 minutes	2	90.7

Lettuce is a vegetable that is commonly eaten raw, and is used for sandwiches and salads. Even though, it is a popular food item, lettuce is not commonly juiced. Those who have tasted this juice, claim that it has easily become one of their favorite vegetable blends. Packed with many essential vitamins and minerals, this juice makes a great lunch or dinner.

Ingredients:
    6 romaine lettuce leaves
    2 oranges

Preparation Instructions:

Wash all the ingredients, then peel the rind off the oranges and cut them into sections. Next chop up the lettuce leaves and place them into the juicer along with the oranges. Make sure the mixture is smooth by juicing on high and enjoy.

Other Health Benefits:

Lettuce is a vegetable that is rich in potassium and dietary fiber. The high amounts of anti-oxidants this juice has contributed to digestive health promoting regularity in the body. Additionally, this vegetable contains lots of nutrition found in vitamin C, vitamin E, vitamin K, iron, potassium, folate, copper, manganese, and phosphorus. Furthermore, lettuce also assists in the improvement of athletic performance and significantly lowers high blood pressure. This vegetable is used to help treat allergic reactions, as well.

Eggplant Orange Juice

Time:	Servings:	Calories:
10 minutes	*1*	*85*

Eggplant is a well-known part of a garden salad or sandwich while blending them into a juice is an uncommon practice. Those who have tried this juice say it is simply amazing. Refreshing and juicy, eggplant juice is one of the healthiest blends that are easily made from home.

Ingredients:
　　1 eggplant
　　2 oranges

Preparation Instructions:

Wash all the ingredients, use a sharp knife to cut off the stem of the eggplant and discard it, then cut the eggplant into sections. Now peel the orange and cut into sections, as well. Add the ingredients to the juicer and drink once it is finished. For the tastiest results add ice.

Other Health Benefits:

Eggplant juice is a diuretic that is high in fiber, protein, and calcium. Contributing to the regulation of the body, and blood pressure, eggplant removes toxins and waste from the body. The benefits of eggplant are mainly found on its skin, which includes vitamins A, C, folic acid, potassium, magnesium, molybdenum and silica. Containing high alkaline levels, zucchini regulates the body's blood pH and neutralizes acidity. As eggplant produces a hormone needed by beta cells during insulin production, it is an effective treatment for diabetes. Eggplant is used to help the immune system, as well as, a form of treatment to fight against cancer.

Blackberry Blend

Time:	Servings:	Calories:
10 minutes	3	74.9

Blackberries are a well-known part of a fruit salad or a parfait. Said to be one of the most delicious drinks, blackberry juice is naturally sweet, and juicy. Packed with many vitamins and minerals, this juice can be consumed any time of the day.

Ingredients:
- 4 cups of blackberries
- 4 tbsp. of honey
- 1 apple
- 1 orange

Preparation Instructions:
Wash all the ingredients. Slice and core the apples and oranges. Now cut them into chunky pieces and begin placing these sections into the juicer, add the blackberries and honey, as well. Mix the blend together briefly and enjoy.

Other Health Benefits:

Blackberries are a natural diuretic that is high in antioxidants, dietary fiber and tannins. Killing bacteria and viruses, blackberries prevent bladder infections and flush out the body. Blackberries contain many nutrients like vitamin E, vitamin A, vitamin C, vitamin K, and vitamin B6, as well as, calcium, manganese, iron, phosphorus and copper. Furthermore, blackberries also contain anthocyanin, an antioxidant plant pigment that contributes to its distinctive color. This fruit has also been used to fight diabetes, urinary tract infection, and anti-aging cosmetics.

Papaya Juice recipe

Time:	Servings:	Calories:
5 minutes	2	124.6

Papaya is best eaten raw or blended into a juice. Said to be one of the most delicious tropical fruits, papaya juice is sweet and refreshing. Packed with many vitamins and minerals this juice is best in the morning as it delivers lots of energy.

Ingredients:
- 2 papayas
- 1 pineapple
- 1 orange

Preparation Instructions:

Wash all the ingredients, then peel off the papaya skin and remove all of the seeds with a spoon. Now place the pineapple on a clean flat surface and cut the top and bottom off so that each side is flat. Now stand the pineapple upright and begin cutting off the rind. Finally, peel the orange and cut it in sections. Lastly add all the fruits to the juicer and enjoy your juice.

Other Health Benefits:

Papayas are high in fiber, calcium, and antioxidants. As a natural diuretic, they are great for the digestive system and for relieving constipation. Stimulating the production of white blood cells, papayas aid the immune system and prevents illnesses. Papayas contain many essential vitamins and minerals like iron, vitamin B6, folate, potassium, and thiamin. Furthermore, papayas have been used to reduce cholesterol. This fruit is also used to treat several other diseases like asthma, arthritis, bronchitis, rheumatism and diabetes.

Grape Blend

Time:	Servings:	Calories:
5 minutes	4	102.1

Grapes are known to many as nature's candy. Said to be one of the sweetest fruits, grapes make the best detox juices as they are tasty and can be used to satisfy sugar cravings. This juice is healthy and is best consumed in the morning or afternoon.

Ingredients:
- 20 baby carrots
- 3 Pears
- 2 cups of grapes

Preparation Instructions:

Wash all the ingredients, then cut and core the pears. Begin placing all of the ingredients into the juicer. Once the juice is in a glass mix it well and enjoy.

Other Health Benefits:

Grapes are high in antioxidants, zinc and dietary fiber. Regulating the digestive system, these fruits can lower blood pressure and prevent overeating. Containing many vitamins and minerals, grapes deliver Vitamin A, vitamin C, alpha and beta carotene, folate, potassium, and manganese. Grapes are used as a remedy against inflammatory diseases, to treat asthma, osteoarthritis and atherosclerosis.

Celtuce Juice Blend

Time:	Servings:	Calories:
10 minutes	1	110.3

Celtuce is a crunchy vegetable that is a combination of stalks and lettuce-like leaves. Usually found in salads, stews, or eaten raw as a snack, this vegetable is known for its bold and robust flavor. Delivering enough energy to last the entire day, celtuce juice can be consumed any time of the day.

Ingredients:
- 2 pears
- 1 large green cabbage
- 1 ginger root
- 1 bunch of celtuce leaves

Preparation Instructions:

Wash all the ingredients, then cut and core the pears. Chop up all of the green cabbage, ginger root, and the celtuce leaves. Peel the ginger by using the edge of a spoon to press across its skin. To reach the skin inside, push the spoon into the folds of the ginger. Now place all of the ingredients inside of the juicer and blend until the texture is smooth. Once the juice is in a glass mix it well and enjoy.

Other Health Benefits:

Celtuce is a vegetable that is rich in folic acid, iron and vitamin C. Celtuce actively regulates the digestive system by regulating bowel movements and softens stools. This vegetable contains many nutritional properties like calcium, magnesium, phosphorus, vitamin A, vitamin B1 and vitamin B2. Enhancing the activity of white blood cells, celtuce contains coumarins which is a class of antioxidants that have been used to fight cancer. Celtuce has been used to treat urinary and gall bladder stones.

Spicy Chili Juice recipe

Time:	Servings:	Calories:
10 minutes	1	134.4

Chili peppers are flavorful vegetables most commonly used to spice up food, in salads, or as a garnish. Known to be one of the most sensational, chili pepper juice is bold and spicy. A great drink for any time of the day.

Ingredients:

    3 carrots
    2 chili peppers
    2 cups of spinach
    2 celery stalks
    1/2 lime
    1 teaspoon of ginger

Preparation Instructions:

Wash all the ingredients, then peel off the lime rind and cut it in half. Peel the ginger by using the edge of a spoon to press across its skin. To reach the skin inside, push the spoon into the folds of the ginger. Now chop up the spinach leaves, peppers and celery stalks. Add the ingredients to the juicer and blend until it is of a smooth consistency.

Other Health Benefits:

Chili peppers contain capsaicin which helps the immune system with its anti-bacterial, anti-carcinogenic, analgesic and anti-diabetic properties. Additionally, chili peppers contain many vital nutrients like niacin, riboflavin, potassium, magnesium, vitamin E, vitamin A, vitamin C, vitamin K, vitamin B6 and manganese. Increasing the metabolism, chili peppers prompt the body to burn calories rapidly. The capsaicin in this vegetable has also been linked to pain relieving qualities, as well.

Crenshaw Melon Juice

Time:	Servings:	Calories:
10 minutes	2	291.1

Crenshaw melons are a hybrid between casaba melons and the Persian melon. A perfect addition to fruit salads or eaten raw, this juice is highly recommended as one of the best tasting drinks available. This juice can be consumed any time of day.

Ingredients:
- 2 apples
- 2 cups of kale
- 2 cups of Swiss chard
- 1/2 Crenshaw melon
- 1/2 cantaloupe

Preparation Instructions:

Wash all the ingredients, then take a sharp knife and peel off the Crenshaw melon skin, as well as, the cantaloupe skin. Cut both of them into small pieces and place to the side. Next, slice open the apple and remove the core. Finally, cut up the kale leaves and the Swiss chard, and begin adding all of these ingredients to the juicer.

Other Health Benefits:

Crenshaw melons are a natural diuretic that are high in antioxidants, fiber and lycopene. Replicating antioxidants, these fruits greatly reduce the effects of destructive oxidant molecules in the body. Crenshaw melons contain many healthy properties like vitamin A, vitamin C, vitamin B6 and potassium. They are also utilized in the treatment of bladder infections, and to flush out the body. Crenshaw melons are considered to be one of the best fruits to use in a detox.

Veggie Apple Breeze

Time:	Servings:	Calories:
15 minutes	8	76.1

Apples make the best snack as they are naturally juicy and sweet. Apple juice is a delicious combination that is sure to satisfy any appetite. This fruit juice can be consumed any time of the day, but is the most beneficial if consumed in the afternoon.

Ingredients:
- 8 carrots
- 4 apples
- 1 cucumber
- 1 inch of ginger

Preparation Instructions:
Wash all the ingredients, then cut and core the apples. Now slice them into pieces that are small enough to fit into the juicer and place them to the side. Chop up the carrots, cucumber and ginger, putting all of the ingredients inside of the juicer. Once the produce is completely juiced mix it with a spoon and drink immediately.

Other Health Benefits:

Rose apples are a diuretic that is high in dietary fiber, pectin and polyphenols. As a natural laxative, apples induce bowel movements, increasing intestinal muscle ability to push toxins out of the gastrointestinal tract. Apples contain many minerals and vitamins like vitamin C, vitamin A, calcium, iron, niacin, and potassium. Apples have significant amounts of flavonoids and phytochemicals that protect cells from damage, reducing the risk of heart disease. Apples have also been used in the treatment of inflammatory diseases.

Cantaloupe Juice recipe

Time:	Servings:	Calories:
5 minutes	3	64.2

Cantaloupe is a species of melon commonly eaten raw or found in fruit salads. Cantaloupe is loved by many, and known for its lightly sweet taste and juicy texture. Delivering many nutritional benefits, this drink is best in the morning, and the afternoon as it delivers high energy and vitality.

Ingredients:
- 2 carrots
- 1/2 cantaloupe

Preparation Instructions:

Wash all the ingredients, then use a sharp knife to peel the rind off of the cantaloupe. Peel and cut the banana into small chunks. Then place all the ingredients inside of the juicer. When the juice is finished, add a few ice cubes and drink it immediately.

Other Health Benefits:

Cantaloupes are fleshy melons that are high dietary fiber, antioxidants, and beta-carotene. Stimulating white blood cells, cantaloupe helps the immune system by killing foreign elements like viruses and bacteria. While delivering many nutrients to the body, this fruit contains folic acid, potassium, vitamin A, vitamin B, vitamin C, niacin, and folate. As a natural diuretic, cantaloupes aids in cleansing out the body, prolonging digestion, and suppressing the appetite. Daily consumption of cantaloupes can reduce the risk of lung disease like emphysema.

Dandelion Delight

Time:	Servings:	Calories:
5 minutes	1	98.3

Dandelions are pesky weeds that are commonly found in stir-fries or salads. Not commonly found in juicing recipes, this weed is surprisingly bold and delicious. Highly recommended for its great taste and many health benefits; dandelion leaves can be consumed any time of day.

Ingredients:
- 3 cups of dandelion leaves
- 1 carrot
- 1 cup of spinach

Preparation Instructions:

Wash all the ingredients, then use a sharp knife to cut the dandelion leaves, carrot, and spinach into small chunks. Then place all the ingredients inside of the juicer. When the juice is finished mix the juice for 1 minute before drinking.

Other Health Benefits:

Dandelion leaves are a multivitamin green that is high in protein, and antioxidants. As a natural diuretic, dandelion leaves remove toxins from the kidneys and the urinary system. Containing many health properties like calcium, magnesium, potassium, manganese, iron, vitamin A, vitamin C, vitamin E, and vitamin B, and zinc. Increasing the absorption of magnesium and calcium absorption, dandelion leaves help the digestive system by improving the growth of healthy bacteria in the body. Dandelion leaves are commonly used in the treatment of bacterial growth in the body.

Bold Lemon Juice recipe

Time:	Servings:	Calories:
10 minutes	2	181.9

Lemons are one of the most popular fruits in the world. Famous for their bold and sour taste, lemons are one of the best juice cleansers available today. Packed with many essential nutrients lemon juice can be consumed any time of the day.

Ingredients:
- 9 tangerines
- 1 lemon
- 1 tsp of ground ginger

Preparation Instructions:

Wash all the ingredients then peel and cut the tangerines and the lemon. Now add all the ingredients to the juicer including the ground ginger. Once the juice is ready, add some ice cubes and drink immediately.

Other Health Benefits:

Lemons are an ellipsoidal yellow fruit that is high in protein, citric acid, and dietary fiber. As a natural diuretic, lemon juice effectively breaks down fat and grease in the stomach, then flushes it out of the urinary and digestive systems. Lemons are very nutritious and contain iron, potassium, magnesium, thiamin, pantothenic acid, vitamin A, vitamin C, and vitamin B6. Containing potent antioxidants called limonoids, lemons strengthen and improve immune system. Used to lower blood pressure and cholesterol levels, lemons neutralize free radicals in the body preventing many forms of cancer.

Sweet Pear Juice

Time:	Servings:	Calories:
5 minutes	1	220.2

Pears are light bulb shaped fruits that are usually eaten raw or in a fruit salad. Known for its sweet and juicy flavor, these fruits make the best juice blends. Delivering many nutritional benefits, pear juice can be consumed any time of day.

Ingredients:
- 1 kiwi
- 1 pear
- 1 celery stalk
- 1/2 of grapefruit
- 1 tbsp of oatmeal
- 1 tbsp of honey
- 6 oz of water

Preparation Instructions:

Wash all the ingredients, then peel and cut the kiwi and grapefruit. The pear has to be peeled, cored and cut while the celery has to be cut down into small chunky pieces. Now begin placing all the ingredients inside of the juicer, including the honey and the oatmeal. Drink up this delicious blend once it's finished.

Other Health Benefits:

Pears are a fruit that is high in dietary fiber, and protein. A natural diuretic, pectin regulates bowel movements while the fructose and glucose deliver lots of energy to the body. A high source of nutrients, pears contain vitamin C, vitamin A, vitamin K, potassium and calcium. Pears have anti-oxidant, anti-carcinogen and glutathione which can prevent high blood pressure or a stroke. Pears are high in boron which helps the body to retain calcium.

Grapefruit Juice

Time:	Servings:	Calories:
7-10 minutes	1	364.1

Grapefruits are large citrus fruits that are usually eaten raw as a snack. Known for its unique taste, these fruits are sweet, bitter and tangy all at the same time. With many nutritional benefits, these juices come highly recommended by many. Great in the morning or the afternoon, this juice delivers enough energy to last the entire day.

Ingredients:
- 3 carrots
- 2 medium apples
- 1 pink grapefruit
- 1 medium beet

Preparation Instructions:

Wash all the ingredients, then peel and cut the grapefruit. The apple has to be cored and cut while the carrots and beets have to be cut down into small chunky pieces. Place all of the ingredients inside the juicer. Drink this nutritious blend once it is finished.

Other Health Benefits:

Grapefruits are high in antioxidants, dietary fiber and beta-carotene. A natural diuretic, this fruit effectively breaks down fat and grease in the stomach, then flushes it out of the urinary and digestive systems. Containing many nutritional properties, grapefruit is a great source of vitamin A, vitamin C, calcium potassium and iron. Producing an alkaline reaction after digestion, grapefruits lower the acid formation in the body. Grapefruits are also used to treat the liver, heart and kidneys.

Pineapple Passion Juice

Time:	Servings:	Calories:
5 minutes	2	155.5

Pineapples are unique fruits, due to its festive composition and rough texture. Pineapple juice is a delicious drink easily made from home and known for its sweet and tangy flavor. Packed with many nutritional benefits, this juice can be consumed during the morning, noon, or night time.

Ingredients:
- 3 oranges
- 2 bananas
- 1/2 of pineapple

Preparation Instructions:

Wash all the ingredients, then place the pineapple on a clean dry surface. Cut off the top and bottom of the pineapple and stand it up. Slice down its side to remove the rind and slice off half of the pineapple and save the rest for another recipe. Peel and cut both the banana and the orange. Now start feeding all of the ingredients into the juicer, blend well and drink immediately.

Other health benefits:

Pineapples are a fruit that is high in dietary fiber, and calcium. Aiding in digestion, the bromelain found in pineapples reduce bloating, constipation, gas, nausea and irritable bowel syndrome. Containing many nutritional benefits like potassium, copper, thiamine, manganese, vitamin B6, vitamin C and manganese, pineapples enable energy production and antioxidant defenses. Great for fighting a cold and the flu, pineapples have natural healing properties that break up mucus and suppress coughs.

Perfect Parsnip Juice

Time:	Servings:	Calories:
5 minutes	1	121.6

Parsnips are a versatile vegetable that can be prepared in an infinite amount of ways. Known for their crunchy robust flavor, parsnips make the best juices. With many vitamins and minerals, this drink is best in the afternoon or evening.

Ingredients:
- 4 Apples
- 2 Parsnips
- 1 teaspoon of nutmeg

Preparation Instructions:

Wash all the ingredients, then cut and core the apples. Now chop up the parsnips and the nutmeg. Place all of the ingredients inside of the juicer and mix it for 1 minute to make sure the contents are mixed properly.

Other Health Benefits:

Parsnips are a vegetable that is high in dietary fiber and protein. A natural diuretic, parsnips regulate the blood pressure and assist in proper nerve function. In addition to helping the immune system, parsnips contain many essential nutrients like folic acid, manganese, potassium, vitamin C and vitamin K. With many antibacterial, antimicrobial and antifungal properties, parsnips stop inflammation in the body. Parsnips have also been used in the treatment of autoimmune and allergic diseases.

Artichoke Vegetable Delight

Time:	Servings:	Calories:
10 minutes	4	214.6

Artichokes are a flower shaped vegetable that are commonly eaten raw, in garden salads, or in stir-fry's. Surprisingly delicious, these vegetables make the best juice as they are high in nutrients. Enjoy this vegetable blend in the afternoon or at night.

Ingredients:

    15 brussels sprouts
    6 Jerusalem artichokes
    6 carrots
    3 cups of green beans
    1/2 lemon

Preparation Instructions:

Wash all the ingredients, then chop up the artichokes, carrots, and green beans. Cut off the artichoke's stem with the base of the artichoke bud. Then pull off the tough dry lower leaves and put into the juicer. Remove the rind from the lemon by peeling the skin and cutting it into a half. Now add all of the ingredients to the juicer and blend for 45 seconds or until the mixture is smooth.

Other Health Benefits:

Artichokes are naturally high in antioxidants, and dietary fiber. As a natural diuretic, this vegetable aids in digestive function, liver function and gallbladder function. Additionally, artichokes contain many essential nutrients like calcium, potassium, niacin, folates, riboflavin, thiamin, vitamin A, vitamin C, vitamin E and vitamin K. With the ability to regenerate tissue, artichokes have long been used to treat ailments in the liver.

Refreshing Mint Juice

Time:	Servings:	Calories:
10 minutes	1	187.5

Mint is an herb that is commonly used as garnish. Surprisingly refreshing and tasty, this herb makes one great juice as it naturally high in many essential nutrients. Drink this blend in the afternoon or evening to add a little freshness to your day.

Ingredients:
- 3 pears
- 1/2 slice melon
- 1 apple
- 4 tablespoons of fresh mint

Preparation Instructions:

Wash all the ingredients, then remove the seeds from the pears and apple, slice in half and take out the cores along with the stems. Use a sharp knife to cut the melon into halves. Scoop out the fiber strings and seeds from the melon by using a teaspoon. Cut the melon into thin cubes to fit into the juicer. Process all of the ingredients into a juicer, stir and serve.

Other Health Benefits:

Mint is an herb that is high in flavonoids, and essential oils. Facilitating digestion, the smell of mint activates the saliva glands in the mouth, which then secretes digestive enzymes. Additionally, the mint is high in many nutrients like iron, magnesium, beta-carotene, calcium, vitamin C and vitamin A. With the natural ability to clear up congestion, mint is used to treat respiratory disorders like asthma or bronchitis. Mint also contains enzymes that have shown to help with cancer treatments.

Sweet Potato Juice recipe

Time:	Servings:	Calories:
5 minutes	1	268.6

Sweet potatoes make the best filling for a pie and the best side to a meal. Naturally sweet and delicious, these vegetables are high in nutrients which is why it is one of the most popular juices to date. Enjoy this sweet sensation in the morning, noon, or night.

Ingredient:

    2 whole grapefruits
    2 sweet potatoes
    1 parsnip
    1 celery

Preparation Instructions:

Wash all the ingredients, then peel and cut the grapefruit. Chop up the sweet potatoes, parsnip, and the celery into small pieces. Then place all of the ingredients into the juicer and blend for 1 minute or until the mixture is a smooth texture.

Other Health Benefits:

Sweet potatoes are vegetables that are high in antioxidants, and beta-carotene. High in dietary fiber, sweet potatoes maintain bowel regularity and movement, preventing constipation. These vegetables contain many healthy properties like vitamin A, vitamin C, iron, and potassium. With the natural ability to ward off cold and flu viruses, sweet potatoes help the immune system by protecting it from free radicals. High in vitamin B6, sweet potatoes reduce the chemical homocysteine in the body which has been linked to the prevention of heart attacks, and degenerative diseases.

Tender Garlic Juice

Time:	Servings:	Calories:
5 minutes	2	204.6

Garlic is a popular herb that is usually cooked into foods. Delivering a burst of robust flavor, this herb makes the best juice as it is high in many essential vitamins and minerals. The best time to enjoy this juice is in the afternoon and the evening as it may be too hard on the stomach in the morning, especially if fasting.

Ingredients:
- 6 carrots
- 6 cups of watercress
- 2 beets
- 2 red onions
- 1 clove of garlic

Preparation Instructions:

Wash all the ingredients, then remove the skin from the garlic, onions, and the beets and cut into a size that is appropriate for the juicer. Next, chop up the watercress and place all of the ingredients into the juicer.

Other Health Benefits:

Garlic is a herb that is high in calcium and vitamin C. Promoting an increase in bile production, garlic helps to lower the fat levels in the liver. Additionally, this juice delivers many nutrients to the body like manganese, phosphorus, selenium, and vitamin B6. Strengthening the body's defense system against allergies, garlic loosens plaque from the artery walls, and regulates blood sugar levels. High in germanium, garlic has been used in the treatment against cancer.

Plum Juice

Time:	Servings:	Calories:
5 minutes	1	253.9

Plums are a purple fruit that is commonly eaten raw or in fruit salads. As one of the most popular blends, this fruit juice offers a sweet and tangy taste. This fruit is high in nutrition and can be consumed throughout the entire day.

Ingredients:
- 6 plums
- 4 apples
- 1 mango

Preparation Instructions:

Wash all the ingredients, then cut and pit the plums and the mango. Slice into pieces that can easily fit inside of the juicer. Next, peel and core the apple, and cut it into four quarters. Now place all of these ingredients into the juicer and blend for 45 seconds. Once the juice is finished, add ice cubes and enjoy it chilled.

Other Health Benefits:

Plums are a fruit that is high in dietary fiber, and antioxidants. Assisting in the production and absorption of iron in the body, plums maintain proper blood circulation throughout the body. Containing many essential nutrients, this fruit is high in vitamin A, vitamin C, beta-carotene, niacin, thiamin and potassium. Consuming plums have also been known to reduce the chances of getting heart disease. Plums also contain anti-carcinogenic properties, which can be used to fight diseases.

Choosing the Best Juicer

While standing in the house wares aisle, it is common to see a juicer and a blender in close range to each other. Kitchen appliances may seem to contain many similarities there many differences one must take into account before purchasing either one. Containing many varied purposes these machines can offer the buyer a wide range of beneficial features.

Juicers are a tool that separates the pulp from fruits, vegetables, and herbs. In this process known as juicing, this appliance removes the juice content from any produce that passes through it. The pulp and fibers gather in one chamber of the juice while sieved juice pours out of the juicer without any fibers in it. Working best with produce that contains a high water content these appliances can easily extract the liquid from the solids. Which then makes the juice easily digestible as there are no fibers to break down. The health benefits of juicing are endless as this process allows the body to absorb all of the nutrients from the produce, and leafy greens without any pieces of fruit or pulp in it. Juicers can make a bunch of healthy foods juices, soups, and salsa.

Blenders are an electronic device that infuses all parts of fruits, and vegetables including the skin, peels, and seeds. Working best with fruits and vegetables that contain both high and low water content, blenders make drinks that are thicker in texture compared to the liquid made from the juicer. When combining the produce into the blender, the drinks are high in fibers, which tend to lock onto nutrients preventing them in some cases from absorbing into the body. As a result, the drinks made from this appliance are thick as there is a significant presence of fibers in it.

Selecting the Juicer

Having a juicer on hand can be a great alternative to purchasing expensive health drinks that may contain unhealthy preservatives. Before buying a juicer, first decide what types of juices can be made using this appliance. Citrus juicers are great for juices that will mainly be made in the morning. For juices that will include a variety of fruits and vegetables than a centrifugal juicer it is best as it easily handles the stems, and seeds found in the produce. Making drinks out of leafy greens and wheatgrass can be an easy task with a masticating juicer as these mechanisms slowly chew the produce. There are several styles of juicers extractors and juicers on the market. Some of them just juice fruits, and vegetables, while others may juice just citrus fruits, or wheatgrass.

Helpful Tips for Purchasing a Juicer

When deciding how much money you're willing to spend on the juicer, consider how much the appliance will be used. For people who are going to be using this appliance every day it is recommended to spend a little extra on some helpful features, like a large feed tube that easily fits whole fruit and vegetables in it.

Make a note of how the appliance is cleaned. Check to see if it is dishwasher safe and if the parts can easily be taken apart and cleaned. Check on how many moving parts the juicer has, the least moving parts it has the easier and faster the clean up. Look for a filter screen and pulp receptacles that are easily removed.

Check on the total speed of the juicer as this is a very important factor in making juice. Fast machines can sometimes be the wrong choice as they are known to heat up while unintentionally killing the enzymes and antioxidants in the juice. Look for a machine that ranges between 3000 RPM and 7000 RPM.

TOP 10 JUICERS

Breville BJE200XL Compact Juice Fountain 700-Watt Juice Extractor

The **Breville BJE200XL** Compact Electric Juice fountain has a durable polymer body that is great for continued use. With its stainless steel filters, this appliance easily juices the pulp with ease. Running on 700-watts the 14,000 RPM motor can juice soft to hard fruits and vegetables. This juicer comes with dishwasher safe parts that can easily be cleaned with no problems

Hamilton Beach Big Mouth Juice Extractor 67650

The **Hamilton Beach 67650A** Big mouth pro juicer comes with an extra large pulp bin that allows for continuous juicing. With an 800 watt motor, this juicer has an 3 inch chute that can easily fit whole vegetables and fruits. This system comes complete with a cleaning brush for the strainer basket and removal parts for dishwashers.

Breville 800JEXL Juice Fountain Elite 1000-Watt Juice Extractor

The **Breville 800JEXL** is a stainless steel juicer that will fit perfectly in any kitchen. This high powered appliance has a 1,300 watt motor that can easily juice 3 whole apples at one time. This juicer can easily be wiped down using an a sponge and some soapy water. A cleaning brush is also provided, as an extra bonus to clean the teeth located inside the juicer.

Breville BJE510XL Juice Fountain Multi-Speed 900-Watt Juicer

The **Breville BJE510XL** Ikon Juice Extractor comes with a stainless steel exterior and black accents. The 5 speed juicing system has 900 watts of power. With the ability to juice an 8 oz. Glass in less than 5 seconds, this juicer has 6,500 (RPM) to 12,500 (RPM). This appliance also comes with removable parts that can easily be placed in the dishwasher.

Breville JE98XL Juice Fountain Plus 850-Watt Juice Extractor

The **Breville JE98XL** two speed juice fountain comes with a heavy-grade polymer exterior. With 850 watts, this juice fountain has a high speed of 12,000 (RPM) to lower speeds at 6,500 (RPM). To clean the micro mesh filter basket, there's a brush and to clean the rest a warm rag or sponge will do.

Omega J8006 Nutrition Center Juicer - Black and Chrome

The **Omega J8006** is a dual stage juicing system that operates at a low speed of 80 RPM. It is through this speed that this appliance delivers the maximum amount of vitamins and nutrients from fruits, vegetables, and leafy greens. This system can easily be washed with a sponge and some warm water.

Omega J8004 Nutrition Center Commercial Masticating Juicer, White

The **Omega J8004** is a masticating juicer that operates at a low speed of 80 RPM, which means there is no clogging, foaming or heat build up within this system. Easy to operate this dual stage juicing system gathers the most nutrients from the produce that its juicing. Running quietly this appliance can be simply wiped down with a warm rag or cloth.

Black & Decker JE2200B 400-Watt Fruit and Vegetable Juice Extractor with Custom Juice Cup

The **Black and Decker JE2200B is a 400-watt juice extractor**. This system can collect 28-Oz of pulp while the pitcher captures 300-ml of freshly squeezed juice. With stainless steel blades, this juicer is dishwasher safe.

Tribest CS-1000 Citristar Citrus Juicer

The **Tribest CS-1000 CitriStar citrus** juicer runs on a 50 watt motor. Extracting the citrus from fruits this juicer has a universal ream that generates the maximum extraction from the large grapefruits to small limes. The powerful and quiet juicer comes with a high clearance spout that prevents clogs for constant juicing operation. Easily clean this with a wet cloth or sponge.

Waring Pro JEX328 Health Juice Extractor

Waring Pro JEX328 runs on a 400 watt motor which generates juice in an instant. The 3 inch feeding chute guarantees that most fruits and vegetables can be placed in the system whole without being cut or sliced. It even comes with dishwasher safe pieces that can easily be disassembled and resembled again.

Some Final Words

Congratulation!

Now you know all TOP 50 Easy Recipes for Juice Fasting. I hope that you have not just enjoyed this book, but also prepared most of these recipes...

I know you could have picked from dozens of books on Juice Fasting. But you took a chance with my book; I hope this book will be according your expectation and help to live healthy.

Before you go, I'd like to say "thank you" for purchasing my book.

1. If you have really enjoyed this book, PLEASE leave a kind review on **Amazon**. As an independent author, word of mouth is only my advertising. You can write your valuable and honest reviews.

2. I know no book is perfect if there are error, omission, or anything you would like to see added or changed please email me at wayofhealthyliving@gmail.com and I promise a quick personal response.

I would love to hear your experience regarding this book

Good Luck!

CPSIA information can be obtained at www.ICGtesting.com
Printed in the USA
LVOW12s1129311213

367567LV00002B/50/P